Cardamom Essential Oil

Benefits, Properties, Applications, Studies & Recipes

by Ann Sullivan

Published in USA by:

Ann Sullivan
217 N. Seacrest Blvd #9
Boynton Beach
FL 33425

© Copyright 2017

ISBN-13: 978-1545429532
ISBN-10: 1545429537

TABLE OF CONTENTS

Introduction

What are essential oils, and how might they be used for therapeutic purposes?

Essential oils are ultra-potent oils, extracted from plants and flowers that have been utilized in medicine for centuries. Presently, they're most commonly used to supplement pharmaceutical medication, but they can also be an effective alternative to pharmaceuticals in the event that you don't have access to them. Before you dismiss essential oils as a means to support the body's natural defenses against injuries and illness, take a look at the historical evidence of the oils' medicinal competence in practice. Your average age-old medical text will demonstrate that essential oils, herbs, and plenty of other natural ingredients have, for thousands of years, successfully enhanced immune function to meet and defeat any number of ailments and injuries. Though traditional medicine is considered "alternative" now, it was once the gold standard. And, frankly, perhaps it still should be, as these natural age-tested remedies can fortify the body's battlements against everything from simple maladies, like headaches, cuts and bruises, to serious diseases, like cancer.

Essential oils are deemed "essential," because the oils are composed of the "essence" of the plant. The difference between essential oils and other oils – like olive oil or vegetable oil, for instance – is that essential oils have high volatility and reduced fixation, which results in faster evaporation, enabling their popular use in aromatherapy. Even at high temperatures, olive and vegetable oils don't evaporate.

Essential oils are especially necessary when it comes to a major natural or man-made disaster or some potential viral outbreak. In these types of dire situations, you may not have quick access (or any access at all) to your standard pharmaceutical supply; so essential oils, along with other alternative medicines, will be your go-to health aids in the case of social collapse, viral outbreak or devastating natural disaster. When medical access is null and void, alternatives to our modern-day standard are the only chance we have to keep pathogens at bay.

You probably don't realize that you already use essential oils every day. They're in perfumes, shampoos, soaps, ointments...they're even used in furniture polish. Why are they found in so many aromatic products? Well, basically, because essential oils are super concentrated aromatic liquids, so their scent is remarkably strong. Let's put this into perspective: to steam tea, you use a few leaves of peppermint or juniper; to produce a single ounce of essential oil, five whole *pounds* of peppermint or juniper leaves are required. Some sources claim that to produce twelve pounds of essential oil would necessitate an acre of peppermint, juniper, or any other oil you're looking to produce en masse. Unlike vegetable oil, you don't often find concentrated therapeutic-grade essential oils sold by the tubload; instead the oils are often sold in easily carried small, dark bottles, perfect for your GOOD bag (Get Out Of Dodge). Which is exactly what this book is aiming to help you do – get out of dodge with your most vital of essential oils intact, in particular a good supply of cardamom essential oil.

Why cardamom, you ask? Well, in order to get you quickly up to speed on this most essential of oils, below we've provided a condensed synopsis of cardamom, after which we'll outline in greater detail the oil's history, properties, and common therapeutic uses, so that you – the consumer – might have a better understanding of the oil's benefits and applications. We've even provided supportive remedies for pure cardamom, as well as blended recipes that incorporate the valuable oil. Chapter 3 will further detail past scientific research on cardamom essential oil.

Now, let's get down to it – **Essential Oil 101: the Basics of Cardamom**.

Summary: Cardamom, or Elettaria cardamomum, has been used for over 3000 years in Ayurvedic and Chinese medicine. The common traditional uses for cardamom were to support the body's defenses against bronchial and digestive issues, but nowadays, it's used to support the body's defenses against everything from indigestion to nausea, from upset stomach to halitosis. The innumerable digestive properties of cardamom are due to its warmth, which bolsters the health of the pancreas, spleen and stomach.

Description: This oil is commonly extracted through steam distillation. The seed is most often used. The oil is clear in color, thin in consistency, and has a medium rich spicy woodsy scent.

Uses: Beyond those applications previously mentioned, additional uses for cardamom essential oil include supporting the body's natural function against colic, halitosis, abdominal inflammation, coughs, dyspepsia, halitosis, debility, flatulence, headaches, sciatica, heartburn, lung infection, pyrosis, sinus infection, vomiting, senility and appetite loss. When it comes to mood and emotion, cardamom can help relieve stress, guilt, shame and fatigue.

Properties: Antioxidant, antiseptic, aphrodisiac, antibacterial, antispasmodic, anticarcinogenic, expectorant, astringent, diuretic, digestive, and stomachic properties.

Application: Dilute 1:1 with a carrier oil. You can apply topically, inhale directly, diffuse or use as a dietary supplement.

Safety Precautions: Cardamom has been approved by the FDA for internal consumption and so can be used as a dietary supplement. No other specific safety precautions were indicated.

Fun facts: In India, Europe and the Middle East, cardamom was often called the "grains of paradise," due to its culinary significance. A prominent 17th century British herbalist, William Cole, even deemed it the "chief of all seeds," because he thought it stacked up protection against nearly any malady.

Chapter 1:
Benefits of Cardamom Essential Oil

Cardamom oil offers a number of therapeutic benefits; but you may be wondering what these benefits are. In this chapter, we'll take a closer look at the history of cardamom and its many uses.

Cultivation of Cardamom

Cardamom, or Elettaria cardamomum, is in the ginger family, Zingiberaceae, and is native to Bhutan, Nepal, India and Pakistan; although, nowadays, Guatemala is one of the largest global cultivators and exporters of cardamom, after it was introduced to the country prior to World War I by the German, Oscar Majus Kloeffer, a coffee planter. Sri Lanka and India are also top cultivators in the modern age, and the spice has become one of the most expensive in the world, with a price per weight just shy of the two global leaders, vanilla and saffron.

Although there are two genuses of cardamom – Amomum and Elettaria – the main type used in producing commercial essential oils is Elettaria, so we will focus on its properties and history. Theophrastus, the Greek "father of botany," actually differentiated between the two cardamoms all the way back in the fourth century BCE. Known as "green cardamom" and "true cardamom," Elettaria cardamomum is found across India through southeast Asia to Malaysia, while Amomum cardamom is found throughout Asia and Australia. The Elettaria genus is a cool and minty spice, while the Amomum genus is a hot spice.

To complicate matters, there are three different primary varieties of cardamom plant – the Mysore, the Malabar, and the Vazhuka. The first is native to Karnataka and produces panicles that grow upwards; the second is native to Kerala and produces panicles that grow horizontally; and the third is a hybrid of the two, producing panicles that grow somewhere in between. Elettaria cardamomum produces small spindly light green seed pods, with tiny black seeds and paper-thin shells.

A History of Cardamom

Derived from the Greek "kardamomon," the word "cardamom" means "cress." This was found in the "Spice" tablets at the House of the Sphinxes in Mycenae; these tablets archived the different flavors of spices. Both genuses were and still are used as food and drink cooking spices.

Due to its strong flavor, cardamom is often found in teas, particularly in the Middle East, and is used frequently in international cuisine. The Middle East utilizes cardamom not only in sweet teas and dishes, but in coffee and savory dishes as well. In India and Nepal, it's one of the most common cooking ingredients, mixed in curries, masalas, and as rice garnishes, while in Finland and Sweden, cardamom is a popular baking spice, incorporated into many sweets, particularly traditional Christmas sweets and breads.

Moreover, the somewhat minty flavor makes cardamom popular to smoke in some areas and has even become an ingredient in chewing gum, such as Wrigley. This is due to the spice's inhibition of halitosis. In fact, throughout the Middle East, the seeds of cardamom are often chewed to rid of bad breath.

Both genuses also have a long history in traditional medicine. In South Asia, cardamom has been used across the centuries in oral hygiene, to target tooth or gum infections and to support the body's natural function against respiratory conditions, such as lung congestion, pulmonary tuberculosis, or throat issues. Furthermore, cardamom has been long popular in aiding digestive issues as well.

Chemical Components

In order to generate the essential oil from the cardamom plant, the seeds must be steam distilled. This results in the oil's key chemical components, which are primarily α-terpineol, myrcene, limonene, menthone, β-phellandrene, 1,8-cineol, heptane and sabinene.

Main Properties of Cardamom Essential Oil

Along with the properties previously mentioned in the introduction, cardamom oil possesses antioxidant, antiseptic, aphrodisiac, antibacterial, astringent, antispasmodic, anticarcinogenic, expectorant, diuretic, digestive, and stomachic properties. With such a versatile range, cardamom is well equipped to fight off any pathogen in the body's path.

Cardamom, as mentioned, is composed of α-terpineol, myrcene, limonene, menthone, β-phellandrene, 1,8-cineol, heptane and sabinene. These components are what instill the enormously beneficial properties within cardamom essential oil. We'll outline these properties below.

Antioxidant

Anything high in antioxidants – whether fruit, beans, or essential oils – is a powerful advocate for your body. Antioxidants both protect against free radicals and repair their damage. What are free radicals? Free radicals are destructive chemicals that invade your body, produced by substances both inside and out. Some free radicals (or oxidants) form through normal bodily reactions, like inflammation, metabolism and aerobic respiration. Other free radicals form outside the body, but enter it due to exposure. These include harmful pollutants, toxins, smoking, drinking alcohol, X-rays, and UV rays, to name a few. Although our bodies produce their own antioxidants, these often become damaged as we grow older; thus, introducing antioxidants into our bodies via essential oils allows these nutrients and enzymes to assist in chemical reactions which destroy the oxidants or free radicals. Cardamom essential oil is a moderate antioxidant, aiming to detox the body of free radicals that lead to disease.

Antiseptic

The antiseptic and disinfectant properties of cardamom essential oil can be reaped topically, applied directly to wounds, or even through burning; the smoke from the oil may destroy airborne germs. Internal use will help keep wounds from becoming infections, while external use will support the inhibition of tetanus. A couple drops of cardamom in water can be used for bathing, as it supports disinfection of hair and skin.

Antibacterial

Cardamom's antibacterial properties make it a powerful protectant against diseases produced by bacteria, such as oral, digestive and urinary tract bacterial infection. What's great is that, unlike some prescription drugs, cardamom has no ill effects on bodily health or on the healthy natural flora that exists within the stomach and intestines. Cardamom is particularly helpful for oral hygiene and halitosis, as it kills bad breath bacteria.

Astringent

An astringent is a chemical compound that shrinks body tissues, which means it can aid skin issues and irritations. Cardamom essential oil benefits everything from skin to hair to gums to muscles to intestines. As an astringent, cardamom is an anti-agent, combatting muscle loss through its ability to strengthen.

Antispasmodic

The antispasmodic properties of cardamom essential oil make it beneficial to such health issues as chronic coughing and other respiratory conditions, along with surgical processes, such as colonoscopy and gastroscopy.

Aphrodisiac

As an aphrodisiac, cardamom can help stimulate sexual arousal, thereby overriding impotence, frigidity, low libido, and erectile dysfunction.

Anticarcinogenic

Cardamom essential oil has been shown to act as an anticarcinogen. An anticarcinogen counters those carcinogens which can potentially develop into cancer. Whereas anticarcinomas are used to support the body's defenses against cancer cells after cancer has developed, anticarcinogenics are natural defenses against the development of cancer.

Expectorant

Throat or respiratory infections can be relieved through the use of cardamom essential oil. Acting as an expectorant, cardamom helps break up and destroy the phlegm and mucus buildup that accompanies sinuses or respiratory infections. Inflamed throat and lungs – and, thus, coughing – can also be relieved through the use of this oil.

Diuretic

If you're looking to lose water weight and reduce blood pressure, cardamom essential oil is your weightloss enhancing agent. The oil stimulates urination, promoting not only the loss of water weight, but the loss of fats, uric acid, sodium, and other body toxins.

Digestive

By boosting the production of absorptive enzymes, the digestibility of nutrients, and the secretion of digestive juices, cardamom essential oil aids the digestive tract significantly, which can make a great impact on the body's overall health by increasing those nutrients absorbed from food.

Stomachic

As a stomachic, cardamom improves stomach function, boosts appetite, and helps to tone the stomach. The oil helps control the stomach's bile, acid and gastric liquids.

Common Medicinal Uses

Used in traditional medicine in the Middle East, cardamom essential oil is safe for consumption or topical application and is most often used to support digestion and stomach issues.

Digestive Aid

A healthy digestive tract means a healthy body, so maintaining good digestion can make a load of difference in how you feel, as a whole. Your digestive tract is between 25 and 30 feet long. If the length of it is not working properly, then there's a chance that food might get caught up and begin to rot within your body. Cardamom effectively supports the digestive tracts natural function by helping induce bile flow throughout the digestive organs, which will benefit your overall health.

Maintaining Health

Overall health can be maintained through the abundance of vitamins and minerals found in cardamom essential oil. The oil contains vitamins B2, B3, and C, and minerals like iron, calcium, potassium, magnesium, manganese, and copper. The potassium helps stimulate cardiovascular health, while iron and copper generate red blood corpuscles. The balancing of these nutrients and the oil's antioxidant properties, boosted by manganese, make cardamom an effective tool in overall health.

Stomach Issues

Cardamom essential oil is beneficial when it comes to stomach issues. Whether you have menstrual cramps, indigestion, nausea or upset stomach, a dosage of this oil and its antispasmodic properties will help ease the pain and uncomfortable nature of these issues.

Oral Hygiene

The antiseptic properties and antibacterial properties of cardamom essential oil help kill bad breath bacteria and also eliminate plaque. The oil also reduces gum bleeding, and maintains the mouth's overall health and cleanliness. Chewing gum oral products contain cardamom for this reason.

Losing Weight

Those who need a boost to lose unwanted weight can use cardamom orally or topically, as it's been shown to reduce water retention. This will eliminate bloating and cut out that bit of extra water weight, and also help rid of toxins in the body and excess fat. The increased urinary function also reduces the chances of urinary tract infections.

Skin Issues

With its antibacterial properties, cardamom essential oil promotes healthy, glowing skin by supporting the body's natural defenses against dry or chapped skin, eczema, dermatitis, acne, and a litany of other skin issues. The high vitamin C content and the oil's antioxidant properties help to detoxify skin, combating bacterial growth while promoting sebum secretion balance within the body. The oil's disinfectant properties also allows for a clean healing process for your skin condition or wound and protects against scarring.

Hair Care

Cardamom essential oil invokes strength, health, and shine in hair follicles, and so is often used as a moisturizing hair tonic. The oil also effectively combats dandruff, so a drop or two in your shampoo can help eliminate this issue. It also serves as a natural highlighter and, when mixed with cinnamon and olive oil or honey, can be applied instead of those chemical colorings.

Safety Precautions & Common Applications

Safety

Some adverse effects may evolve when using pure essential oils. Some essential oils should not be used when pregnant, for example, as they may cause miscarriage. Allergic reactions, too, may occur, especially when applied topically. Always administer an allergy test before committing fully to topical administration. When used with other medications, essential oils may react negatively. If you are on any current prescription medications or have a chronic illness, such as high blood pressure, epilepsy or liver disease, then researching the effects of essential oils against your own personal medical history will eliminate any potentially problematic issues.

Cardamom has been approved by the FDA for internal consumption and so can be used as a dietary supplement. No other specific safety precautions are indicated. Dilute 1:1 with a carrier oil. You can apply topically, inhale directly, diffuse or ingest.

Blends

Oftentimes, essential oils are manufactured as blends of several pure oils. For instance, doTerra's On Guard Essential Oil Blend is a mix of cinnamon, clove, rosemary, and eucalyptus. This blend can be used to boost the immune system to help support the body's defenses against colds, viruses and flus. The downside to blends is that the more oils added to the mix, the higher the probability your patient may react negatively to the blend if he/she is prone to allergies. There is also the possibility of phototoxicity when working with blends.

Regardless of these possible effects, essential oils are a viable option for support the body's defenses against a number of conditions. Those looking to support the body's defenses against or maintain their own personal health, or that of their family's, should become educated on the uses of essential oils, their natural remedies and the methods of administration. Only then can you begin building your kit of essential oils for survival.

Chapter 2:
Recipes for Cardamom Essential Oil

In this chapter, we'll offer various recipes for cardamom essential oil, both for pure cardamom supportive remedies and blends. For pure supportive remedies, we've provided the appropriate application and dosage to help your body's natural function address specific ailments, from appetite loss to skin issues. When it comes to blends, herbalists and aromatherapists often combine cardamom essential oil with, orange, rose, cinnamon, bergamot, cloves, cedarwood, and caraway. We'll offer some fantastic supportive blending options in the second half of this chapter.

Pure Supportive Remedies

Anger

Calm anger, stress or nerves by diffusing cardamom essential oil throughout the home. You can also dilute in a 1:1 ratio with a carrier oil and apply topically in a full-body massage.

Appetite Loss

If grief, stress, illness, or depression causes you to experience appetite loss, diffuse cardamom essential oil throughout the home or dilute in a 1:1 ratio with a carrier oil and massage over the stomach, then cup your hands around your nose and inhale. You can also place a drop in your drinking water.

Asthma

To combat asthma, dilute cardamom essential oil in a 1:1 ratio with a carrier oil, then to open up airways, apply topically by massaging over the chest and into the reflex points of the feet during an asthma attack. You can also diffuse throughout the home or inhale directly to help stave off attacks.

Bacterial Infections

Take down bacterial infections by diluting cardamom essential oil in a 1:1 ratio with a carrier oil and applying topically over the affected area or into the reflex points of the feet. You may also place a few drops in a bath or diffuse the oil for a similar effect.

Bronchitis

Support the body's natural defenses against bronchitis by diluting cardamom essential oil in a 1:1 ratio with a carrier oil, then apply topically, massaging into the throat, chest and back. Additionally, you can steam two drops of cardamom essential oil in a pan of water, remove the steaming pan from the stove, pour into a bowl, place a towel over your head and inhale. You can also place a drop of oil onto your shirt collar for effective application throughout the day or inhale directly.

Congestion

Clear congestion by diluting cardamom essential oil in a 1:1 ratio with a carrier oil, then apply topically, massaging it over the affected area. Additionally, you can steam two drops of cardamom essential oil in a pan of water, remove the steaming pan from the stove, pour into a bowl, place a towel over your head and inhale. You can also inhale the oil directly for nasal congestion, or diffuse throughout the home.

Cough

Relieve coughs by diluting cardamom essential oil in a 1:1 ratio with a carrier oil, then apply topically, massaging it over the throat, chest and back, as well as into the reflex points in your feet. You can also diffuse throughout the home to help relieve those suffering from coughing and help protect those who are healthy.

Diarrhea

If you're experiencing diarrhea, cardamom essential oil is the answer. Apply topically by diluting the oil in a 1:1 ratio with a carrier oil and massaging it into the abdomen in a counterclockwise motion, or place a drop of the oil in your drinking water throughout the day.

Digestive Support

Cardamom aids the digestive tract and can be taken orally or topically. Place a drop into your drinking water for internal administration or dilute the oil in a 1:1 ratio with a carrier oil and apply topically to the abdomen in a clockwise motion and into the reflex points of the feet. You can also diffuse throughout the home.

Edema

To relieve edema, dilute cardamom essential oil in a 1:1 ratio with a carrier oil and massage the solution into the affected area, toward the heart.

Emotional Balance

Maintain mood balance by diffusing cardamom essential oil throughout the home. If making concentrated efforts to stave off mood swings, inhale directly for 30 seconds or more throughout the day. You can also apply topically, diluting cardamom in a 1:1 ratio with a carrier oil and massaging over the body's energy centers.

Flatulence

Relieve gas by applying cardamom essential oil to the abdomen in a clockwise rotation. You can also place a drop in a glass of water and take orally.

Food Poisoning

Strengthen your body's natural defenses against food poisoning by adding a drop of cardamom to your drinking water. You can also inhale directly or apply topically, diluting cardamom essential oil in a 1:1 ratio with a carrier oil and massaging it into the abdomen.

Frustration

Frustration can be calmed by diffusing cardamom essential oil throughout the home or office.

Halitosis

Cardamom essential oil can target bad breath both by eliminating the bacteria that produces the odor and by providing your mouth a fresh scent. Either administer orally by adding a drop to drinking water or apply a drop directly to the tongue or to your toothbrush before your regular oral hygiene regimen.

Headache

Headaches can be relieved with cardamom oil by inhaling directly, diffusing the oil throughout the room or, for a more direct application, dilute cardamom essential oil in a 1:1 ratio with a carrier oil and apply topically over the area of pain. Avoid the eyes.

Indigestion

Cardamom aids the digestive tract and can be taken orally or topically. Place a drop into your drinking water for internal administration or dilute the oil in a 1:1 ratio with a carrier oil and apply topically to the abdomen in a clockwise motion and into the reflex points of the feet. You can also diffuse throughout the home.

Infections

To fight off infections, you can dilute cardamom essential oil with a carrier oil and apply topically to the affected area or to the soles of the feat. You can also diffuse throughout the room, whichever application is more appropriate to your specific infection.

Inflammation

Calm inflammation and provide lymphatic system support by diluting 1 or 2 drops of cardamom essential oil in a 1:1 ratio with a carrier oil, then apply topically, massaging it over the affected area towards the heart.

Invigorating

Invigorate and stimulate body function by diffusing cardamom essential oil throughout the home, inhaling directly, or adding a drop to your meal.

Muscles Aches

To relieve sore muscles, dilute cardamom essential oil in a 1:1 ratio with a carrier oil and massage the solution into the affected area, toward the heart.

Muscle Spasms

Reduce muscle spasms by diluting cardamom essential oil in a 1:1 ratio with a carrier oil and massaging the solution into the affected area, toward the heart.

Nausea

To stave off or relieve nausea, apply a single drop of cardamom essential oil to a piece of cloth or on the shirt collar to be inhaled when feeling nauseous. You can also take internally, applying a drop to a glass of drinking water.

Respiratory Support

To fight respiratory issues, dilute cardamom essential oil with a carrier oil and massage over the chest and neck. You may also apply a drop beneath the nose or diffuse the oil for a similar effect.

Stomach Spasms

Reduce stomach spasms by diluting cardamom essential oil in a 1:1 ratio with a carrier oil and massaging the solution into the affected area, toward the heart. You can also take internally, adding a drop to a glass of drinking water.

Ulcers

Target ulcers internally by placing a drop in each meal or glass of water, or externally by diluting cardamom essential oil in a 1:1 ratio with a carrier oil and applying topically, massaging into the stomach and into the reflex points of the feet.

Uplifting

To uplift the spirit, diffuse cardamom essential oil throughout the home or apply topically, diluting cardamom in a 1:1 ratio with a carrier oil and massaging over the chest.

Vomiting

To inhibit vomiting, place a drop of cardamom essential oil in your drinking water and take internally. You can also inhale directly, diffuse throughout the home, or apply topically, diluting cardamom in a 1:1 ratio with a carrier oil and massaging over the abdomen.

Blends

Abdominal Cramp Rub

Ingredients

- 6 drops Roman Chamomile Essential Oil
- 7 drops Cardamom Essential Oil
- 2 drops Angelica Root Essential Oil
- 3 ounces Sweet Almond Oil

Directions

To relieve abdominal cramps, combine all ingredients in a small jar or bowl. Mix thoroughly. Massage over the stomach as needed.

Abdominal Cramp Rub II

Ingredients

- 4 drops Roman Chamomile Essential Oil

- 4 drops Cardamom Essential Oil

- 4 drops Angelica Root Essential Oil

- 6 drops Clary Sage Essential Oil

- 30 mL Marula Oil

Directions

To relieve abdominal cramps, combine all ingredients in a small jar or bowl. Mix thoroughly. Massage over the stomach as needed.

Aphrodisiac Massage Blend

Ingredients

- 4 drops Sandalwood Essential Oil

- 4 drops Jasmine Essential Oil

- 2 drops Cardamom Essential Oil

- 2 drops Rose Oil

- 15 mL Marula Oil

Directions

To stimulate sexual desire, combine all ingredients in a small jar or bowl. Mix thoroughly. Apply in a full-body massage.

Body Massage

Ingredients

- 1 drop Cardamom Essential Oil
- 2 drops Cinnamon Essential Oil
- 2 drops Jasmine Essential Oil
- 4 drops Myrrh Essential Oil
- 6 drops Ginger Essential Oil
- 1 ounce Sweet Almond Oil
- 1 ounce Jojoba Oil

Directions

Combine all ingredients in a bottle. Tighten the lid and shake well. Massage over body, but not into sensitive areas. Shake well before each use.

Constipation Relief

Ingredients

- 5 drops Black Pepper Essential Oil

- 5 drops Cardamom Essential Oil

- 15 drops Patchouli Essential Oil

- 2 Tbsps Sweet Almond Oil

Directions

In a small bowl or container, mix all ingredients until well combined. Massage in a clockwise motion into the lower abdomen. Also massage into the shoulders, neck and back.

Muscle Pain

Ingredients

- 4 drops Cardamom Essential Oil

- 4 drops Ginger Essential Oil

- 4 drops Wintergreen Essential Oil

- 1 Tbsp Sweet Almond Oil

Directions

To create a massage oil for muscle pain, combine all ingredients in a small container, mixing until well blended. Keep covered and shake before each use.

Uplifting Scent

Ingredients

- 1 drop Ginger Essential Oil

- 2 drops Clove Essential Oil

- 2 drops Cassia Essential Oil

- 3 drops Cardamom Essential Oil

Directions

For an uplifting spicy chai fragrance, combine all ingredients in a diffuser and diffuse throughout the home.

Chapter 3:
Cardamom Essential Oil Studies

Many studies have been done on essential oils to discover and prove their therapeutic qualities. In the case of the great number of cardamom studies, many of the properties attributed to the essential oil (noted in this book and elsewhere) are quite often validated through the scientific research of accredited universities and published by accredited scientific journals. In this chapter, we'll discuss a small portion of these studies. It's important to note that research on essential oils is constant and evolving. Keep up with any recent research, as it may turn up even further valuable uses for these miracle oils.

Study 1 – Cancer Chemopreventive Potential

In this study published by the Asian Pacific Journal of Cancer Prevention, the cancer chemopreventive potential of cardamom essential oil were examined, with the following results: "Cardamom (Elettaria cardamom), also known as 'Queen of Spices', has been traditionally used as a culinary ingredient due to its pleasant aroma and taste. In addition to this role, studies on cardamom have demonstrated cancer chemopreventive potential in in vitro and in vivo systems. Nevertheless, the precise poly-pharmacological nature of naturally occurring chemo-preventive compounds in cardamom has still not been fully demystified. In this study, an effort has been made to identify the proapoptopic, anti-inflammatory, anti-proliferative, anti-invasive and anti-angiogenic targets of Cardamom's bioactive principles (eucalyptol, alpha-pinene, beta-pinene, d-limonene and geraniol)...This study revealed vital information about the poly-pharmacological anti-tumor mode-of-action of essential oils in cardamom. In addition, a probabilistic set of anti-tumor targets for cardamom was generated, which can be further confirmed by in vivo and in vitro experiments."

In summary, this study attempted to target cardamom's anti-tumor properties and which compounds of cardamom affected such properties. The study obtained a list of the target proteins which are associated with various cancers and examined the factors associated with anti-tumor activity. The study found that cardamom's eucalyptol bound to Caspase 3, a protein which plays a key role in the execution-phase of cell apoptosis, or programmed cell death, which demonstrates the part cardamom may play in the cytotoxicity of cancer cells.

Reference
http://www.ncbi.nlm.nih.gov/pubmed/23886174]

Study 2 – Insecticidal Properties

In this study published by the Journal of Insect Science, the insecticidal effects of cardamom essential oil were examined, with the following results: "Use of insecticides can have disruptive effects on the environment. Replacing the chemical compounds in these insecticides with plant materials, however, can be a safe method with low environmental risk. In the current study, chemical composition and insecticidal activities of the essential oil from cardamom, Elettaria cardamomum L. (Maton) (Zingiberales: Zingiberaceae) on the adults of three stored product pests was investigated...These results suggest that essential oil of E. cardamomum is a good choice for control of stored product pests."

The study examined cardamom essential oil's effects on the bruchid beetle, (Callosobruchus maculatus Fabricius), the red flour beetle (Tribolium castaneum Herbst), and the flour moth (Ephestia kuehniella Zeller). Native to the UK, the bruchid beetle, also known as the "bean weevil," infests various types of seeds and beans, often living inside them. Of Indo-Australian origin, the red flour beetle is a global pest found in food grains and other stored products, like pasta, cereal, beans and nuts. The flour moth is a pest native to the Mediterranean and India and, of course, infests flour.

After testing cardamom against these three pests, the study found that the flour moth was highly sensitive to the oil's insecticidal properties. It was also highly effective against the bruchid beetle and more mildly effective against the red flour beetle. This activity demonstrates cardamom's potential as a natural insecticide against these three product pests.

Reference
http://www.ncbi.nlm.nih.gov/pubmed/22242564]

http://www.ncbi.nlm.nih.gov/pmc/articles/PMC3281396/

Study 3 – Nausea

In this study available on PubMed, the effects of cardamom essential oil were examined, with the following results: "Postoperative nausea (PON) is a common complication of anesthesia and surgery. Antiemetic medication for higher-risk patients may reduce but does not reliably prevent PON. We examined aromatherapy as a treatment for patients experiencing PON after ambulatory surgery. Our primary hypothesis was that in comparison with inhaling a placebo, PON will be reduced significantly by aromatherapy with (1) essential oil of ginger, (2) a blend of essential oils of ginger, spearmint, peppermint, and cardamom, or (3) isopropyl alcohol. Our secondary hypothesis was that the effectiveness of aromatherapy will depend upon the agent used...The hypothesis that aromatherapy would be effective as a treatment for PON was supported. On the basis of our results, future research further evaluating aromatherapy is warranted. Aromatherapy is promising as an inexpensive, noninvasive treatment for PON that can be administered and controlled by patients as needed."

This study aimed to assess the efficacy of a blend of essential oils – including cardamom, ginger, spearmint and peppermint – on nausea postanesthesia care. 301 subjects were analyzed, and were asked to provide a description of their level of nausea on a 0-3 scale, after which they were provided either the blend, ginger on its own, or isopropyl alcohol. The study found that the reduction in the level of nausea significantly decreased when provided the blend (P < 0.001) and ginger (P = 0.002), and the amount of antiemetic medications requested afterward decreased significantly as well. This demonstrates the potential of cardamom in a blend as an antidote to nausea.

Reference & Photo Credit:
http://www.ncbi.nlm.nih.gov/pubmed/22392970]

Study 4 – Sporicidal & Antibacterial Properties

In this study available in the Journal of Microbiology & Biotechnology, the sporicidal effects of cardamom essential oil were examined, with the following results: "Alternative methods for controlling bacterial endospore contamination are desired in a range of industries and applications. Attention has recently turned to natural products, such as essential oils, which have sporicidal activity. In this study, a selection of essential oils was investigated to identify those with activity against Bacillus subtilis spores...Our data have shown that essential oils exert sporicidal activity and may be useful in applications where bacterial spore reduction is desired."

Bacillus subtilis is a Gram-positive bacterium with a high tolerance of extreme environmental conditions. Though found in average human gut commensal, B.subtilis has the potential to cause disease in immunocompromised individuals and, on very rare occasions, food poisoning.

In this study, the sporicidal activity of thirteen essential oils, including cardamom, were examined against B.subtilis. Cardamom was found to be one of the most effective, demonstrating its antibacterial and sporicidal potential.

Reference & Photo Credit:
http://www.ncbi.nlm.nih.gov/pubmed/20075624]

http://www.jmb.or.kr/journal/viewJournal.html?year=

Study 5 – Antimicrobial Properties

In this study published by the BMC Complementary and Alternative Medicine, the antimicrobial effects of a cardamom essential oil species were examined, with the following results: "The main objective of this study was the phytochemical characterization of four indigenous essential oils obtained from spices and their antibacterial activities against the multidrug resistant clinical and soil isolates prevalent in Pakistan, and ATCC reference strains... cardamom (Amomum subulatum)...was analyzed on GC/MS...Among all the tested essential oils, oil from the bark of C. verum showed best antibacterial activities against all selected bacterial strains in the MIC assay... Cinnamaldehyde was identified as the most active antimicrobial component present in the cinnamon essential oil which acted as a strong inhibitory agent in MIC assay against the tested bacteria. The results indicate that essential oils from Pakistani spices can be pursued against multidrug resistant bacteria."

In summary, this study showed that cardamom oil was effective as an antibacterial agent against pathogenic strains Salmonella typhi (D1 Vi-positive), Salmonella typhi (G7 Vi-negative), Salmonella paratyphi A, Escherichia coli (SS1), Pseudomonas fluorescens and Staphylococcus aureus. Salmonella strains can cause an array of illnesses from typhoid fever to food poisoning. E. coli, as well, often results in serious food poisoning. Though a rare bacteria, P. Fluorescens may target those with compromised immune systems, such as cancer patients. And, lastly, S. aureus causes a whole host of illnesses and infections, including Staph infections, pimples, boils, impetigo, carbuncles, abscesses, scalded skin syndrome, and even pneumonia or meningitis.

Cinnamaldehyde, one of the main chemical components in Pakistani spices, including cardamom, was found to be the most active prohibitory agent against these strains.

Reference
http://www.ncbi.nlm.nih.gov/pubmed/24119438]

http://www.ncbi.nlm.nih.gov/pmc/articles/PMC3853939/pdf/1472-6882-13-265.pdf]

Study 6 – Anti-carcinogenic and Anti-mutagenic

In this study available on PubMed, the anti-carcinogenic and anti-mutagenic effects of cardamom essential oil were examined, with the following results: "The influence of essential oils from naturally occurring plant dietary items such as cardamom, celery seed, cumin seed, coriander, ginger, nutmeg, and zanthoxylum on the activities of hepatic carcinogen-metabolizing enzymes (cytochrome P450, aryl hydrocarbon hydroxylase, and glutathione S-transferase) and acid-soluble sulfhydryl level was investigated...Our observations suggest that intake of essential oils affects the host enzymes associated with activation and detoxication of xenobiotic compounds, including chemical carcinogens and mutagens."

The study showed that cardamom essential oil, in particular, significantly reduced hepatic enzyme activities. Hepatic enzymes increase the amount of carcinogens and toxins within the body. Cardamom's effect on this enzyme demonstrates that it may be effective in managing the levels of xenobiotic compounds in the human body. Xenobiotic compounds are foreign chemical substances which are not naturally found within the body, such as pollutants, chemical carcinogens and mutagens.

Reference & Photo Credit:
http://www.ncbi.nlm.nih.gov/pubmed/8072879]

Chapter 4:
The Ins & Outs of Essential Oils

Where do essential oils come from?

Plants and plant species naturally produce essential oils for various reasons, one being to draw pollinator insects to them, another being to repel invading organisms (bacteria, animals). A number of chemical compounds compose each plant's essential oil, and the combination of these compounds is specific to each oil, which then instills in the oil its own unique properties. Essential oils can be harnessed from all sorts of plant components, including flowers, leaves, bark, fruit, roots, and resin. For instance, cinnamon oil is harnessed from bark, lemon oil from the peel, and lavender oil from lavender flowers. Certain plants can produce a few chemical variants of the same essential oil, which are acquired from different parts of the plant. Some of these parts produce a large amount of oil, while others produce just a smidgen. The oil's quality and potency depends upon a number of factors, including the subspecies of the plant, its soil conditions, the time of year and even the time of day you harvest it.

How are essential oils extracted?

Essential oils can be extracted from plants through various methods, including pressing, distillation, solvent and maceration. Let's take a brief look at each:

Pressing Method

Commonly used with citrus fruit, the pressing method extracts the oil through a technique which involves pushing the fruit peels through a press. Oily fruits and plants are best suited for this technique. Orange oil, for example, is extracted from orange skins through the pressing method.

Distillation Method

This technique harkens back to the days of old-timey moonshiners, as the same sort of method used to create strong liquor can be used to extract essential oils. Using a still, boiled water and plant materials will create steam which is then cooled by coils and condensed into a combination of water and oil. This combination doesn't mix, so the oil can then be extracted from it.

Solvent Method

Through a multi-step process, certain plant and flower oils can be extracted using alcohol and other solvents, which extort the essential oil from the plant materials.

Maceration Method

When a "carrier" or fixed oil or lard is mixed with the plant material and set out in the sun, over a period of time, the carrier oil is infused with the plant's essence. Heat sources, other than the sun, are often used to speed the process. Throughout the process, more plant material is added to produce a more potent oil.

How do you use essential oils?

Although some studies about the effectiveness of essential oils are conducted by small companies or even individuals, a number of them are conducted by the food and cosmetic industries. In general, the pharmaceutical industry shows next to no interest in herbal medicine, primarily because there are few options to patent such products. Being as such, the product's lack of profitability results in a lack of research funding. Regardless, the historical uses of essential oils tell us what we need to know: these oils have been effectively administered for centuries. The therapeutic qualifications of essential oils can be plotted in the survival of the human race across cultures and generations.

Another reason that studies on essential oils have not resulted in much conclusive evidence as to their overall effectiveness is because definitive results are sometimes difficult to prove, as the quality of each batch of oil can vary for a number of reasons. One is that essential oils are impossible to standardize. As mentioned above, even the slightest variance in soil conditions and the time of harvesting – as well as innumerable other factors – will produce a different product quality and potency. In addition, essential oils are often obtained from various species of the same plant; Eucalyptus radiata and Eucalyptus globulus can both be used in the making of therapeutic-grade eucalyptus oil and, as a result, they may have slightly different properties and degrees of strength or effectiveness.

Just as there are a number of methods by which to extract essential oils, there are a number of methods to administer them therapeutically. The variety of chemical compounds in each essential oil means that their benefits and applications also vary across the board. Below are a few of these methods.

Topical Administration

Direct application of many essential oils works like a sponge, as skin sops up chemicals and other things (like sunlight, for instance). Topical application is best when you want to clear up an ailment on the skin's surface or in the underlying muscle tissue. When applying topically, you may either massage the oil into the skin or simply dab on the skin for therapeutic results. You might combine the essential oil with a carrier oil for topical use in order to dilute its potency. This is safer, as the oil is so concentrated. You may support your body's defenses against rash or muscle pain in this manner, but you should always test your patient for allergies before applying. Adverse effects are produced by natural chemicals as much as synthetic ones; poison ivy, for example.

To test for allergens, place a drop or two on your patient's inner forearm. If a rash develops within 12 to 24 hours, then the patient is allergic. In addition, phototoxicity – sun exposure resulting in an exacerbated burn – may be an issue when citrus oils are applied topically. So one must proceed with caution when applying essential oils using this method.

Inhalation Therapy

Commonly known as "aromatherapy", this essential oil application is effective for inner ailments, like sore throat or cold. In a steaming bowl of distilled or sterilized water, add a few drops of essential oil and, with a towel over your head, bend over the bowl and inhale. The towel captures the vapors, making the technique even more effective. Essential oils can also be placed in a diffuser or potpourri throughout a room to produce somewhat diluted therapeutic effects.

Ingestion

When using this method, proceed with caution. Direct ingestion of essential oils must be monitored and applied in small doses that are diluted in a tablespoon or more of any carrier oil – olive oil, for example. If you are unsure of dosage amounts, make a tea with the relevant herb instead. Although the effects of this diluted use may be weaker, this application is a better alternative than an overdose of essential oils.

What are the general benefits of using essential oils?

Replacement for Prescription Drugs

One practical benefit for using essential oils is, of course, their substitutive nature; they can replace Rx drugs, which is the ultimate reason to educate yourself on their administration and to begin stockpiling your essential oil supply. One of the potential threats of economic or social collapse is the lack of resources, and primarily the inability to procure prescription drugs. Being as such, finding suitable supplements should be a priority when preparing for the worst.

Their portability is also a major bonus when it comes to survival prepping. The fact that these ultra-concentrated oils take up little-to-no space makes toting them to your shelter all the simpler should the need arise. And, because essential oils are highly concentrated, the application used in most methods of administration requires only a drop or two of oil, which means that tiny bottle will be long-lasting.

Cost Effective Supplement

Though money may be the last thing on your mind when it comes to prepping for a survival situation (money may even be obsolete in the event of social collapse), it is worth noting that the expense of essential oils pales in comparison to prescription drugs. Essential oils are a cost effective supplement to prescription medicine.

No Expiration Date

Another benefit of essential oils is that they do not expire, neither do they have "proper storage" requirements. A number of medicines and medicinal products must be replaced every couple years, so this sets essential oils ahead of the pack when it comes to shelf life.

Versatility

Essential oils also offer great versatility. Apart from providing therapeutic benefits, essential oils can be repurposed for household and hygienic applications. For instance, if you're looking for something that might serve your dental hygiene needs in a time of crisis, the protective oil blend is your go-to essential oil. If you want to maintain your skin's tone and condition, frankincense and lavender will do the trick; the latter also serves as sunscreen, so you can inhibit sun damage as well.

When it comes to the house or shelter, you can use essential oils to deodorize, which will come in handy in a disaster scenario where things might start to smell fishy due to lack of proper utilities and care. For example, after the 2011 tsunami and the subsequent nuclear reactor meltdown in Japan, a nurse named Risa Nakahira used essential oils to deodorize and sanitize putrid public bathrooms in overpopulated evacuation facilities. As relief workers searched for survivors, often wading through debris and decay, Nakahira also deodorized their boots and masks using essential oils. The possibilities of these natural oils are endless.

They are also versatile when it comes to the range of patients they're capable of supporting. The wellness of everyone from your great grandfather to your infant baby can be fortified with the aid of essential oils in the appropriate dosage. They even come in handy when supporting the wellness of livestock or pets. From teething infants to dementia in the elderly, from teenagers with acne to dogs with urinary tract infections, essential oils can serve any patient with nearly any ailment.

Conclusion

Now that you know all about what cardamom essential oil can do for you – where it originates, how it's extracted, its benefits and properties, and the different methods of administration – you can use it confidently to support the body's defenses against health issues and start to assemble a kit of essential oils for survival. Essential oils can be purchased online or at your local holistic treatment store.

The various benefits of essential oils and their properties are countless. To build your own kit, first focus on acquiring the essential oils which may bear more relevance to your health issues or the potential health threats within your environment. When it comes to skin health, for instance, myrrh essential oil will be one of your more crucial oils, due to its antibacterial, anti-inflammatory, antifungal, and astringent properties.

Used as a supplement or as your go-to for immune system support, blood circulation, or gum and hair health, the application of myrrh essential oil in medicine has survived for centuries and will survive centuries more. When it comes down to it, you don't need to rely on pharmaceuticals; essential oils, herbs, and plenty of other natural ingredients can be used to help support any number of health issues, whether ailment or injury.

Essential oils are essential to your survival in the case of viral outbreak, social collapse or natural disaster because, when the SHTF, your access to pharmaceuticals will likely either be limited or eliminated altogether. Alternatives to our modern-day standard will equate survival when no other option exists. And when it comes to a life-or-death situation, you can't let your health decline, no matter the state of the world.

DISCLAIMER AND/OR LEGAL NOTICES: Every effort has been made to accurately represent this book and it's potential. Results vary with every individual, and your results may or may not be different from those depicted. No promises, guarantees or warranties, whether stated or implied, have been made that you will produce any specific result from this book. Your efforts are individual and unique, and may vary from those shown. Your success depends on your efforts, background and motivation.

The material in this publication is provided for educational and informational purposes only and is not intended as medical advice. The information contained in this book should not be used to diagnose or treat any illness, metabolic disorder, disease or health problem. Always consult your physician or healthcare provider before beginning any nutrition or exercise program. Use of the programs, advice, and information contained in this book is at the sole choice and risk of the reader.